Prevent and Beat Cancer

Naturally Healing Through Alternativep Treatments and Optimal Nutrition Strategies

By

Dr Mark Rainey

Disclaimer

The information provided in this book is for educational and informational purposes only. The author, Dr Mark Rainey, is not a medical professional, and the content presented should not be considered as a substitute for professional medical advice, diagnosis, or treatment.

Readers are encouraged to consult with qualified healthcare professionals regarding their individual health concerns. The author and publisher disclaim any liability for the decisions made by readers based on the information provided in this book.

The content in this book reflects the author's research and understanding at the time of writing. Health-related information is subject to constant evolution, and readers are advised to verify the latest developments and consult relevant sources.

The author and publisher do not endorse or promote specific products, treatments, or therapies mentioned in this book. Any mention of such products or services is for informational purposes only and does not constitute an endorsement.

Individual results may vary, and the author and publisher are not responsible for any adverse effects or consequences resulting from the implementation of suggestions or recommendations presented in this book.

By reading this book, readers acknowledge and agree to the terms of this disclaimer. If you do not agree with these terms, it is advised not to rely on the information provided in the book.

For any specific health concerns or questions, readers are advised to seek guidance from qualified healthcare professionals. Always consult with a healthcare provider before making changes to your diet, lifestyle, or medical treatment plan.

The author appreciates the readers' understanding of the limitations inherent in providing general health information and encourages a proactive and informed approach to individual health and well-being.

Table of contents

Introduction

As we navigate the complexities of health, cancer frequently arises as a significant obstacle. However, it's crucial to view it beyond mere villainy. It's akin to unraveling a sophisticated language, and this book serves as our roadmap into that intricate realm.

Cracking the Code of Cancer

Consider cancer not merely as a foe but as a message – an indication that there's something amiss in the intricate choreography of our body's metabolism. It's akin to interpreting the underlying narrative within our cells, discerning a tale of disarray and disturbance.

This isn't your conventional health manual. It's an expedition that veers away from the conventional routes, unveiling the metabolic mysteries underlying the presence of cancer. It's a venture into uncharted territories where fresh perspectives and opportunities emerge.

Here, we're crafting a healing narrative that diverges from the conventional storyline. We're integrating strands of unconventional therapies and the profound influence of nutrition. Each chapter serves as an entry point, a chance to equip ourselves with insights that transcend the conventional wisdom.

Think of this book as an enticement to delve into the essence of comprehending cancer. Let's traverse alternative routes of healing together, guided by the language of nutrition. It's an expedition where our goal isn't just to overcome an ailment; we're striving for a realm where health and vitality thrive. Let's embark on this collective journey toward healing and enlightenment.

1

Digging into the Heart of the Matter

Visualize our body as a complex and elaborate garden, a vibrant canvas where the narrative of cancer gradually reveals itself. To gain a comprehensive understanding, we must delve deep into the soil, where the intricate roots of this multifaceted issue originate. Cancer isn't merely a stroke of misfortune; it's about comprehending the terrain that cancer inhabits and thrives within.

Genetic Soil

Our genes serve as the architectural plan for this garden. Just as various soils yield different results, inherited genetic variations can predispose individuals to specific types of cancer. However, this awareness isn't a definitive fate; it's a guidebook. Armed with this knowledge, we can chart and potentially modify the trajectory. It's akin to having privileged insights, enabling us to customize our strategies for both prevention and treatment.

Environmental Influences

Our garden isn't an entity unto itself; it exists within a broader environment, continually engaging with external forces. Pollution, stress, and other external factors function much like weather patterns, shaping the health of our garden. We'll delve into how these elements affect our internal terrain, either fostering a nurturing environment for well-being or creating conditions conducive to cancer growth.

Lifestyle Choices

Every day, we sow seeds in our garden. Our dietary preferences, physical activity levels, and sleep habits – each decision influences the overall ambiance of our garden. It's akin to choosing whether to cultivate vibrant flowers or inadvertently nurture weeds. We'll delve into how our daily decisions impact our garden, recognizing the significance of our dietary intake, physical exertion, and sleep quality in this ongoing interplay.

Consider this: the food we consume serves as nourishment for our garden, exercise functions as a workout session for the soil, and sleep provides crucial downtime for the garden's rejuvenation. These choices elevate us from passive inhabitants to proactive gardeners, tending to our well-being with purposeful action.

The Tapestry of Roots Unveiled

As we traverse the intertwining paths of genetics, environment, and lifestyle, a profound revelation emerges. Cancer isn't merely a solitary chapter; it's a continuous narrative influenced by our decisions, genetic predispositions, and environmental surroundings.

This journey isn't solely about unraveling the origins of cancer; it beckons us to actively participate in the ongoing saga of our well-being. Empowered with this understanding, we assume the role of garden architects – nurturing the soil, mitigating potential risks, and cultivating seeds of resilience.

2

The myths about cancer

Navigating the realm of cancer treatment is akin to venturing into a labyrinth of intricacies, where misconceptions and realities intertwine, influencing the path to recovery. Join us as we embark on this journey, untangling prevalent myths surrounding conventional cancer treatments and illuminating the truths that navigate us through this complex landscape.

Myth: One Size Fits All in Cancer Treatment

You may have encountered the notion of a universal remedy for addressing cancer, but the reality is far more nuanced. Cancer is inherently diverse, mirroring the individuality of those it afflicts. While conventional therapies such as chemotherapy and radiation hold significant efficacy, their impact hinges on variables like cancer type and stage. Tailoring treatment strategies to align with the unique attributes of both the cancer and the patient is paramount for achieving positive outcomes.

Myth: Conventional Treatments Are the Only Option

A common misconception suggests that traditional methods are the sole path to recovery. However, the realm of cancer treatment is expansive and constantly progressing. Integrative methodologies, blending conventional treatments with complementary therapies, are increasingly acknowledged for their capacity to improve holistic wellness throughout treatment. It entails discovering a harmonious blend tailored to individual needs and preferences.

Myth: Treatment Means Saying Goodbye to Quality of Life

A misconception persists that embracing conventional cancer treatments equates to sacrificing one's quality of life. While these treatments undoubtedly pose challenges, it's worth noting that advancements in supportive care have made significant strides. Effectively managing side effects and prioritizing overall well-being are fundamental aspects of contemporary cancer care. It's not solely about survival; it's about experiencing a meaningful and enriching life throughout and beyond treatment.

Myth: Natural Remedies Can Replace Conventional Treatments

The appeal of natural remedies can sometimes perpetuate the misconception that they have the capacity to supplant conventional treatments. It's important to dispel this notion – while lifestyle adjustments and holistic methods can certainly enhance treatment, they are not intended to replace conventional approaches. The key lies in integration, cultivating a harmonious relationship between conventional treatments and natural strategies. Your healthcare providers are equipped to assist you in navigating this balance effectively.

Truth: Treatment Decision-Making Is a Personalized Process

Here's a fundamental truth that warrants widespread recognition: the process of making decisions about cancer treatment is deeply individualized. It entails a thorough comprehension of your particular circumstances – the specific type of cancer you're confronting, its distinct attributes, and your overall well-being. Collaborative decision-making between you and your healthcare providers is paramount. It's your body, your health, and your narrative. Engaging actively in these conversations guarantees that your treatment approach is customized to your needs.

Truth: Conventional Treatments Have Evolved Significantly

The landscape of conventional cancer treatments has undergone substantial progress. There has been remarkable advancement, particularly with targeted therapies and immunotherapies taking center stage. These cutting-edge methods strive to improve treatment efficacy while mitigating adverse effects. Keeping abreast of these breakthroughs enables you to play a proactive role in deliberations concerning your treatment regimen. Indeed, being well-informed is empowering.

Truth: Emotional and Mental Well-being Are Integral to Treatment

Let's delve into the emotional ups and downs frequently encountered during the cancer journey. While conventional cancer treatments focus on addressing the physical aspects of the illness, it's essential to recognize the significance of emotional and mental well-being. Supportive care, counseling, and integrative therapies all play pivotal roles in a comprehensive approach. This entails nurturing resilience, discovering coping strategies, and acknowledging the profound link between mental and physical health.

3

Path to healing

Hello! Let's delve into a topic that's likely at the forefront of your thoughts – your well-being. It's a journey filled with twists and turns, much like navigating a winding road. So, let's equip ourselves with a symbolic map and embark on this exploration of medical advice and treatment options together.

The Guides on Your Journey
Initially, let's highlight the importance of your healthcare team, akin to a knowledgeable group of guides. This team comprises doctors, specialists, and other healthcare professionals, each bringing a wealth of expertise to the table. Feel free to rely on them, inquire, and actively

participate in decision-making. They're here to assist you in navigating this journey effectively.

Understanding Your Diagnosis

Upon receiving a diagnosis, it's akin to pinpointing the beginning of your expedition. Your healthcare provider assumes the role of a storyteller, elucidating the specifics of your condition – its nature, current stage, and prospective treatment options. This information forms the bedrock for charting your individual path towards improved health.

Treatment Options

Let's delve into treatment possibilities – the varied routes in this healthcare terrain. There exist traditional approaches such as surgery, chemotherapy, and radiation, alongside emerging methods like immunotherapy and targeted treatments. It's akin to possessing a spectrum of tools in a toolkit. Complementary and alternative therapies introduce additional layers, addressing not just the physical but also your emotional and mental wellness.

Being the Captain of Your Ship: Informed Decision-Making

Taking an engaged role in decision-making is akin to piloting your vessel. Armed with insights about your diagnosis and treatment alternatives, you assume the helm of your healthcare expedition. Engage in transparent discussions with your healthcare team, explore second opinions if necessary, and assess how each choice resonates with your principles and way of life.

Navigating Challenges

As you navigate through this voyage, obstacles may arise. That's perfectly normal – this is where supportive care steps in. Mitigating side effects, tending to emotional health, and embracing palliative care are akin to possessing a dependable compass and toolkit to steer through the more challenging stretches of the expedition.

Staying Updated

The realm of healthcare is akin to a flowing river, continuously shifting and advancing. Keeping abreast of fresh treatments, clinical studies, and breakthroughs empowers you. Your healthcare team serves as your informational hub, updating you and directing you towards potential avenues that resonate with your health objectives.

Lifestyle Choices

Apart from medical treatments, lifestyle serves as the daily toolbox for well-being. Factors like nutrition, physical activity, stress management, and sleep all contribute. Engage in discussions with your healthcare team regarding how your lifestyle can enhance your treatment strategy. The goal is to weave these daily choices into the broader canvas of your health journey.

Building Your Team

Your healthcare team isn't merely a collection of specialists; they're your companions aboard this journey. Establishing a strong partnership entails open communication, mutual regard, and collaborative decision-making. Regular updates ensure that your plan adapts according to your responses and evolving requirements.

4

Your mindset can beat cancer

Sure, let's delve into something significant – the mindset for overcoming cancer. It's more than just a slogan; it's an attitude that can truly impact your journey towards well-being. So, picture us having a conversation, and let's explore how you can nurture a mindset prepared to confront any challenge.

Let's dissect it. The beat cancer mindset isn't about denying reality; it's about cultivating mental resilience, positivity, and a firm belief in your ability to navigate adversity. It's a mindset that declares, "I'm confronting this directly, and I possess the strength to overcome."

Let's start by clarifying: adopting a beat cancer mindset doesn't entail suppressing your emotions. It's about facing them head-on, acknowledging the fear, uncertainty, and perhaps anger, alongside moments of joy and gratitude. It's about embracing the full spectrum of emotions while maintaining inner strength.

Now, let's discuss perspective. Having a beat cancer mindset requires a shift – transitioning from feeling trapped or powerless to recognizing that you hold agency. You're not merely a bystander; you're actively charting the course toward healing.

Maintaining a positive outlook is akin to fueling the engine of your beat cancer mindset. It's not about denying reality; it's about deliberately directing your attention towards the positives, the opportunities, and the silver linings. It's choosing to see the bright side even amidst challenges.

Additionally, setting intentions is like charting your course on a mental map. It involves determining your objectives for each day, each treatment, and your overall path to healing. These intentions serve as your guiding lights, offering direction even when the way forward appears uncertain.

In the journey of cultivating this mindset, your mental support network acts as your pit crew. Surround yourself with encouraging individuals—friends, family, and healthcare providers—who contribute positive energy. They're the ones rooting for you, emphasizing that you're not navigating this path solo.

Now, let's delve into the mind-body connection. Techniques such as meditation, visualization, and mindfulness extend beyond mere relaxation; they serve as avenues to harness the potency of your mind for holistic wellness and resilience.

It's akin to attuning yourself to the synergy between your thoughts and your physical well-being.

In the mindset geared towards conquering cancer, each incremental progress counts as a triumph. Whether it's completing a treatment, overcoming a challenging day, or discovering a glimmer of happiness, these achievements serve as the foundation of your resilient mindset.

Flexibility is equally vital in fostering this mindset. It involves remaining adaptable amidst the shifts—in treatment strategies, emotional responses, and daily rituals. Envision your mindset as a navigator constantly recalibrating the sails, steadily progressing towards the destination of healing.

Here's the crux of it all: Your mindset serves as a superhero cape throughout your battle with cancer. The beat cancer mindset revolves around you—your distinct inner strength and your unwavering dedication to resilience each day. When obstacles arise, your mindset becomes the rhythm, the pulsating force that drives you onward. By nurturing this mindset, you're already paving the way toward triumph.

5

Anti-cancer diet

Let's delve into something truly influential: your dietary choices. But we're not just discussing any diet here; we're delving into the realm of an anti-cancer diet. Consider it more than a mere compilation of foods; it's a dietary approach that can authentically bolster your overall health. Take a seat, and let's dissect how the items you choose to include on your plate can serve as a guide toward a healthier version of yourself.

What's Behind the Anti-Cancer Diet?

What's all the talk about an anti-cancer diet? It's not about imposing stringent limitations; it's about incorporating foods onto your plate that act like miniature superheroes, packed with essential nutrients and antioxidants. These foods aren't just delicious; they're your body's partners in promoting good health.

Visualize your plate as a canvas, with fruits and vegetables serving as the vibrant hues of paint. The more diverse the colors, the better! Each shade delivers a variety of nutrients and antioxidants, nature's method of providing your cells with a boost. So, indulge in that rainbow of goodness.

Embrace whole grains; they're the underrated champions of your diet. From brown rice to quinoa and oats, they're rich in fiber. Fiber not only promotes digestive health but also helps stabilize blood sugar levels, making it a dynamic duo for gut health.

Proteins are the foundation of life, and opting for lean sources is essential. Fish, poultry, legumes, and nuts are your top picks for essential amino acids without excess saturated fats, providing your cells with the necessary building blocks.

While not all fats are harmful, the anti-cancer diet highlights the beneficial ones. Omega-3 fatty acids, present in fish, flaxseeds, and walnuts, act as superheroes combating inflammation and creating an unfavorable environment for certain cancers.

When it comes to meats, moderation is key, particularly with processed and red meats, as excessive consumption has been associated with higher cancer risk. It's not about complete avoidance but rather about mindful consumption and considering how frequently they feature in your diet.

Water plays a vital role silently supporting your health. Staying hydrated is crucial for various bodily functions, including digestion, circulation, and detoxification. It's akin to providing your cells with a revitalizing drink to ensure they remain in optimal condition.

Watch out for added sugars, as they can be stealthy troublemakers associated with inflammation and obesity, which may increase the risk of cancer. Be diligent about checking labels and reducing consumption of sugary beverages and snacks. Opt for natural sugars from fruits as a healthier alternative.

Transform your kitchen into a natural pharmacy with herbs and spices like turmeric, garlic, ginger, and green tea. These ingredients not only enhance flavors but also contain compounds that discourage the proliferation of cancer cells, essentially saying, "You're not welcome here!"

If you enjoy the occasional drink, that's alright. However, as with many things, moderation is essential. Excessive alcohol consumption has been associated with an increased risk of certain cancers, so it's important to find a balance.

In the broader context, adopting an anti-cancer diet isn't merely following a set of rules; it's embracing a lifestyle. It involves appreciating the natural bounty that surrounds us, selecting foods that nurture your body, and transforming each meal into a masterpiece of health. Your plate transcends mere sustenance; it becomes a canvas, and every bite becomes a brushstroke contributing to the portrait of a healthier, more vibrant you.

6

Empowering Your Body

Envision your body as a fortress, with nutrition serving as the commander directing operations. Essential nutrients derived from your diet function as a disciplined army, safeguarding against potential threats, particularly cancer. It's not just about consuming food; it's about equipping your body with the resources necessary to fortify its defenses.

Enter the frontline defense: antioxidants. Present in fruits, vegetables, and whole grains, these formidable agents neutralize free radicals – rogue elements capable of harming your cells and potentially triggering cancer. It's akin to possessing a shield that deflects harmful assaults.

Additionally, plant-based phytochemicals are nature's elite forces, strategically embedded within plants. They aren't merely ornamental; each possesses unique properties that aid in cancer prevention and management. Therefore, every vibrant fruit and vegetable incorporated into your diet serves as a recruitment of these specialized forces, enhancing your body's defense mechanisms.

Moreover, prioritize fiber intake. Acting as the post-battle cleanup crew, fiber, abundant in whole grains, fruits, and vegetables, assists your body in eliminating waste and toxins. A well-maintained battlefield is less conducive to the proliferation of cancer cells, and fiber ensures efficient movement to maintain optimal conditions.

Essentially, Omega-3 fatty acids emerge as the champions against inflammation. Present in fatty fish, flaxseeds, and walnuts, these beneficial fats establish a bodily environment less susceptible to chronic inflammation, a factor associated with cancer onset.

Immune-Boosting Nutrients
Your immune system functions as your army, and specific nutrients serve as reinforcements. Nutrients such as vitamin C, vitamin D, and zinc play vital roles in bolstering your immune response, akin to generals ensuring your troops are prepared for defense.

Healthy Microbiome
Within the complex ecosystem of your gut, you have supporters – your microbiome. A diet abundant in fiber and fermented foods fosters a thriving microbiome. These beneficial bacteria not only assist in digestion but also help regulate inflammation and bolster overall immune function, fortifying your body's defenses.

Maintaining a Healthy Weight

Maintaining a healthy weight isn't solely about aesthetics; it's a tactical advantage in the war against cancer. Excess weight, particularly concentrated around the midsection, is linked to an increased likelihood of specific cancers. Adopting a well-rounded diet and engaging in regular exercise become your partners in this combat.

Reducing Processed Foods

Processed foods, abundant with sugars, unhealthy fats, and additives, can act as adversaries in your defense plan. They not only fuel inflammation but also disrupt your body's intricate equilibrium. Limiting their consumption bolsters your defensive line.

Hydration: The Essential Supply Line

Imagine hydration as the lifeline to your fortress. Remaining adequately hydrated is vital for all bodily functions, ensuring that your body's defense mechanisms operate smoothly and are prepared to confront any challenges that arise.

In the war against cancer, your diet becomes your armory. Every meal is a strategic maneuver, and your plate serves as the battleground where the struggle for your health unfolds. By selecting a variety of nutrient-dense foods, avoiding harmful substances, and upholding a healthy lifestyle, you empower your body to withstand potential threats with resilience. Here's to the potent weapon that is nutrition – your ally in the quest for a healthy, cancer-resistant existence.

7

The new body

Hey, let's pause for a moment to explore something truly fascinating – the remarkable ability of your body to heal itself. It's akin to having a covert team of superheroes constantly at work, ensuring your well-being remains optimal. So, let's venture into the captivating realm of your body's innate healing prowess.

1. Cellular Repair: Have you ever pondered how your body rebounds from a bruise or a cut? Well, it operates with an impressive repair mechanism at the cellular level. Imagine miniature worker cells meticulously repairing and replacing damaged ones, ensuring your body undergoes continuous self-renewal.

2. Inflammation: Inflammation goes beyond mere redness and swelling; it's your body's rallying call against potential dangers. When there's an injury or infection, it acts as an alarm, indicating, "Attention, repairs are needed!" It marks the dynamic start of the healing journey.

3. Immune Vigilance: Your immune system? Absolute superheroes. White blood cells, antibodies – they constitute this formidable team guarding your body, poised to eliminate any intruders. It's akin to having an elite security force dedicated to maintaining your peak health.

4. Blood Circulation: Consider your blood vessels as akin to Amazon delivery trucks, but instead of packages, they transport nutrients, oxygen, and immune cells. This circulatory network serves as your vital link, ensuring that every corner of your body receives the necessary supplies crucial for healing. It's like having an incredibly efficient delivery service at your disposal!

5. Hormonal Harmony: Hormones function as conductors directing a harmonious symphony of healing within your body. In times of urgency, stress hormones take the stage, while growth hormones play a pivotal role in tissue repair. Together, they form a precisely coordinated ensemble, ensuring that your body responds appropriately to various situations.

6. Neurological Influence: Surprisingly, your mind takes center stage in this narrative. The intricate relationship between mind and body entails your nervous system impacting immune reactions and releasing neurotransmitters. It's akin to a dynamic collaboration between your mental state and physical health.

7. Regeneration and Scar Tissue: As the healing process unfolds, regeneration and scar tissue formation become active participants. Regeneration strives to return tissues to their original form, while scar tissue intervenes when the situation demands resilience. It's akin to your body weaving a tapestry of restoration, adjusting to various adversities along the way.

8. Restorative Sleep: Have you ever marveled at the rejuvenating power of a restful night's sleep? During deep sleep, your body unleashes growth hormone, initiates tissue repair, and strengthens the immune system. It's akin to hitting a reset button each night, ensuring your internal healing mechanisms are fully energized when you wake up.

9. Nutrient Support: Your body relies on essential nutrients to sustain its ongoing healing processes. Think of vitamins and minerals as the building blocks for cellular repair, immune function, and overall health. Consequently, your diet plays a pivotal role in providing your body with the necessary tools for its healing toolkit.

10. Psychological Resilience: The role of your mental and emotional well-being in the healing process should not be overlooked. Stress and negativity can hinder healing progress, acting as obstacles, while maintaining a positive mindset serves as a motivational catalyst, empowering your body to confront and overcome challenges with resilience.

8

Detoxification

Okay, let's delve into the fascinating domain of detoxification and its crucial significance in the process of recovering from cancer. It's more than just a trendy term; it's a fundamental mechanism that can greatly influence your body's capacity to heal. So, get comfortable, and let's delve into the profound link between detoxification and the journey to cancer recovery.

Detoxification resembles giving your body a thorough cleanse, working at the cellular level. Imagine it as a meticulous process where cells purge waste and toxins, paving the way for a rejuvenated start. This internal purification is vital for establishing a milieu where your body can prioritize healing.

Enter the liver, the body's primary detox orchestrator. This powerhouse organ metabolizes and detoxifies substances, ensuring that harmful compounds are transformed into less toxic or water-soluble forms for expulsion. Upholding liver health becomes pivotal in the detoxification-cancer recovery nexus.

In our contemporary environment, we encounter an array of environmental toxins, ranging from pollutants to pesticides. Detoxification assumes a critical role in eliminating these potentially harmful substances from your system, lessening the overall burden on your body and fostering a more favorable setting for recovery.

Detoxification goes beyond mere toxin elimination; it also enhances nutrient absorption. A purified, detoxified system absorbs vital nutrients more effectively, supplying the necessary energy for the intricate healing process, especially during cancer recovery.

Oxidative stress, stemming from an imbalance between free radicals and antioxidants, is associated with cancer development. Detoxification bolsters your body's antioxidant defense mechanism, mitigating oxidative stress and fostering a cellular milieu less conducive to cancer advancement.

Your gut serves as a pivotal player in detoxification. A thriving gut microbiome facilitates efficient detox processes, aiding in substance breakdown and bolstering overall digestive health. This interdependent relationship between gut health and detox holds particular significance in cancer recovery efforts. Detoxification transcends mere physical cleansing; it encompasses mental and emotional well-being. Stress, a recognized cancer catalyst, can be alleviated through practices such as meditation and mindfulness, forming a comprehensive detox approach that supports your holistic recovery journey.

While detox diets garner attention, lifestyle choices significantly influence the detoxification process. Regular physical activity, proper hydration, and sufficient sleep all contribute to optimal detoxification, reinforcing your body's capacity to rebound from cancer-related challenges.

Chronic inflammation is a recognized instigator in cancer onset and advancement. Detoxification, by curbing the overall toxic burden, aids in inflammation management. It serves as a soothing agent, fostering an environment less conducive to cancer cell proliferation.

Understanding that detoxification isn't a universal solution is crucial. Tailoring approaches to individual health conditions, identifying specific toxins, and addressing the distinct demands of cancer recovery guarantee that detox plans are attuned to your body's needs.

9

Role of exercise in Healing cancer

Let's delve into a significant aspect of cancer recovery – the role of exercise. It's not just about physical activity; it's about understanding how each movement can profoundly impact your body and spirit. So, get comfortable, and let's discuss why exercise is a key component of the journey toward healing from cancer.

Exercise serves as a boost for your immune system. It activates your body's defense mechanisms, increasing the production of immune cells and antibodies, which stand ready to combat cancerous cells. It's akin to transforming your immune system into a vigilant superhero team, always prepared for action.

Imagine this scenario: Regular exercise acts as a catalyst, promoting circulation throughout your entire body, ensuring each cell receives a fresh influx of oxygen. Oxygen is akin to the lifeblood for your cells, maintaining their vitality and establishing an inhospitable environment for cancer cells.

Furthermore, exercise serves as a regulator for hormonal balance. It aids in weight management by burning calories and maintaining hormone equilibrium. This equilibrium ensures that everything remains in proportion, making it challenging for cancer cells to infiltrate.

Moreover, chronic inflammation can stir up trouble, but exercise has the remarkable ability to mitigate its effects. It operates like a cooldown session post-workout, dampening inflammation and fostering an environment where cancer cells encounter obstacles in their persistence.

Recovery encompasses not only physical well-being but also mental health. Exercise acts as a catalyst for releasing endorphins, those natural mood boosters that transform your workout into a therapeutic session. It's as if your body is reaffirming, "We've got this!" even amidst the most challenging moments.

Furthermore, quality sleep is invaluable during the recovery process, and exercise facilitates its attainment. While you're in dreamland, your body engages in significant repair work, addressing the aftermath of the hurdles posed by cancer.

Although cancer treatments can deplete your strength, exercise acts as your body's repairman. It aids in rebuilding what has been broken down, fostering a sense of resilience and empowerment. It's akin to sending a message to cancer, stating, "We're regaining strength, stronger than before."

Navigating through treatment side effects can be daunting, but exercise steps in as your reliable ally, alleviating the burden of these challenges. It's akin to having a steadfast companion by your side in the arena, empowering you to confront treatment with resilience and determination.

Moreover, engaging in group exercise or activities goes beyond the physical workout; it fosters social connection. It's like being surrounded by understanding friends who offer encouragement, creating a supportive community that infuses positivity into your healing journey.

Furthermore, it's essential to recognize that exercise isn't a one-size-fits-all solution. It's about finding what resonates with you. Whether it's a leisurely stroll in the park, dancing freely in your living room, or embracing the tranquility of a gentle yoga practice, the choice is yours. Tailoring exercise to suit your preferences ensures that it becomes a nurturing companion in your individual path to recovery.

10

Usefulness of pomegranate

Let's explore the remarkable benefits of pomegranates and their role as a health champion, particularly in the fight against cancer.

To start, pomegranates act as a formidable shield for your body. They're brimming with antioxidants, such as punicalagins and anthocyanins, which serve as guardians against harmful free radicals. These antioxidants defend your cells, shielding them from potential damage that could lead to cancer. Essentially, they provide a protective barrier, safeguarding your body from the daily stresses it encounters.

Furthermore, pomegranates possess remarkable anti-inflammatory properties, akin to skilled firefighters tackling chronic inflammation. Inflammation is often depicted as the antagonist in this narrative, but pomegranates have the ability to quell its intensity. By reducing inflammation, they create an inhospitable environment for cancer cells, dampening their ability to thrive. It's akin to dialing down the intensity of a gathering where cancer cells thrive, disrupting their preferred habitat.

Moreover, pomegranates exhibit a superhero-like ability to induce cell self-destruction. They may signal cancer cells to undergo apoptosis, a process where these rogue cells essentially commit suicide. This action is pivotal in halting the spread of cancer, preventing it from metastasizing to other parts of the body. It's analogous to instructing errant cells to retreat, effectively impeding the progression of cancer.

Let's delve into another layer of pomegranates' prowess: their ability to impede the growth of tumors by blocking their access to blood supply. Tumors rely on a steady blood flow for nourishment and growth, but pomegranates intervene, saying, "Not so fast." Compounds like ellagic acid found in pomegranates can inhibit the formation of new blood vessels, which tumors depend on for sustenance. It's akin to severing their supply line, stalling their progression.

Additionally, pomegranates serve as mediators in the hormonal landscape. Certain cancers thrive in environments of hormonal imbalance. Pomegranates step in as peacekeepers, aiding in the regulation of hormones, particularly estrogen. By maintaining hormonal equilibrium, they mitigate the risk of hormone-related cancers. It's like restoring order to prevent cancer-promoting hormonal disruptions.

Furthermore, envision pomegranates as guardians of your cellular blueprint, your DNA. DNA, the genetic blueprint of your cells, requires safeguarding. Pomegranates, armed with antioxidants, assume the role of protectors, shielding your DNA from mutations and harm. It's akin to donning a superhero cape, fortifying your genetic code against potential damage and preserving its integrity.

Elevating your immune team is another remarkable attribute. Pomegranates serve as cheerleaders for your immune system, rallying immune cells into action and ensuring a robust defense force. It's akin to having a vigilant army poised to repel any health threats that dare to intrude.

They also play the role of janitors within your body. Pomegranates aid in detoxification, acting as diligent cleaners, eliminating toxins and waste. A cleaner internal environment reduces strain on your body's defenses, allowing them to focus their energy on combating potential cancer risks.

While not directly related to cancer, maintaining a healthy heart is paramount. Pomegranates offer an added benefit by promoting cardiovascular health. A strong and healthy heart provides a solid foundation for confronting various health challenges, including cancer.

And let's not overlook their delectable appeal. Whether enjoyed as crunchy seeds, refreshing juice, or flavorful additions to recipes, incorporating pomegranates into your diet adds a delightful dimension to harnessing their anti-cancer properties.

Therefore, envision pomegranates as your flavorful companion in the battle against cancer. While they aren't a miraculous cure, integrating them into your meals represents a delicious stride toward a lifestyle that nurtures your body's defense mechanisms. Here's to the small yet potent pomegranate!

11

Optimizing Your Diet Based on Methylation

Let's simplify the concept of methylation and its relationship with diet without delving into a scientific textbook.

So, what exactly is methylation? It's a biochemical process where a small cluster of atoms known as methyl groups attaches to various molecules in your body. Why is this significant? Because it acts like a backstage director, impacting functions such as DNA regulation, neurotransmitter production, and aiding in detoxification.

Now, how do you eat to make this methylation thing work smoothly?

1.Load up on Leafy Greens:

Consider kale, spinach, and similar dark leafy greens. They're abundant in folate, a B-vitamin that plays a crucial role in methylation, acting as the star player in ensuring your body functions seamlessly.

2.Say Hi to B12:

Animal products like meat, fish, and eggs are rich sources of B12, which also contributes to methylation. If you prefer plant-based options, you can opt for B12-fortified foods or supplements to ensure you're meeting your body's needs in this biochemical process.

3.Beet It for Betaine:

Beets, whole grains, and spinach contain betaine, which acts as a supportive donor of methyl groups, aiding in the methylation process.

4.Chow Down on Choline:

Eggs, liver, and broccoli are rich in choline, a nutrient that facilitates methylation, providing your body with the necessary resources for efficient methylation processes.

5.Riboflavin Richness:

Almonds, mushrooms, and dairy products are sources of riboflavin (B2), which supports the function of folate, aiding in efficient methylation. It's akin to ensuring seamless collaboration within the methylation team.

6.Fishy Friends and Flaxseeds:

Omega-3 fatty acids found in fish, flaxseeds, and walnuts act as facilitators, promoting a favorable environment for methylation processes to occur smoothly.

7.Magnesium Matters:

Leafy greens, nuts, and whole grains contain magnesium, acting as the support team for enzymes, ensuring that the methylation process proceeds smoothly behind the scenes.

8.Turmeric Tidbits:

Curcumin, found in turmeric, is believed to promote methylation. Incorporating turmeric into your cooking adds not just flavor but also enhances your methylation efforts, adding a tasty boost to the process.

9.Steer Clear of Processed Stuff:

Processed foods aren't ideal for methylation since they often lack essential nutrients and may contain additives that disrupt the process. Opting for whole foods is akin to recruiting the A-team for your methylation journey, ensuring you have the necessary ingredients for success.

Keep in mind, your individuality matters: Each person is distinct, influenced by genetics and health status. If you're delving into the intricacies of methylation, consult with a professional—whether a trusted healthcare provider or a registered dietitian. They can provide personalized insights tailored to your specific requirements.

12

Herbal Treatments for Malaria Kills Cancer Too

Okay, let's discuss herbs – the vibrant greens that could potentially play a role in fighting cancer.

1. Turmeric:

Have you ever come across turmeric? It's that bright yellow spice commonly found in kitchens. What's fascinating is that it contains curcumin, which certain studies suggest could inhibit the growth of cancer cells. Moreover, it boasts powerful anti-inflammatory properties.

2. Green Tea:

Green tea isn't just a soothing drink; it's loaded with catechins, potent antioxidants. Certain studies indicate that these compounds could potentially hinder the growth of cancer cells and may even reduce the likelihood of certain types of cancer.

3. Mushrooms:

The mushrooms commonly used in stir-fries, like reishi and shiitake, are gaining recognition for their possible abilities to enhance the immune system and inhibit tumor growth.

4. Ginger:

Apart from its reputation for soothing upset stomachs, ginger contains gingerol, which some research suggests could inhibit the growth of cancer cells. Ginger might just surprise you as a potential ally in the fight against cancer.

5. Astragalus:

In traditional Chinese medicine, astragalus is regarded as a potent supporter of the immune system, acting as a superhero to bolster the body's defenses against various illnesses, including cancer.

6. Milk Thistle:

Introducing milk thistle, recognized for its supportive role in liver health. With its component silymarin, scientists are investigating its potential in cancer prevention and treatment. Consider it as a protective shield for your liver, standing guard against harm.

7. Artemisinin (Sweet Wormwood):

Artemisinin, extracted from sweet wormwood, is emerging as a contender worth noting. While some research suggests its potential in targeting cancer cells, there's still much to learn about its mechanisms and effectiveness.

8. Frankincense:

Indeed, the substance often linked to ancient practices, frankincense contains boswellic acids, which studies suggest could possess anti-inflammatory and anti-cancer properties. It's akin to a historical combatant against cancerous cells.

9. Cannabis:

You're likely familiar with it. Components found in cannabis, such as THC and CBD, aren't solely for recreational purposes. They're demonstrating potential in alleviating cancer-related symptoms. Certain studies even discuss their potential in combating cancer itself.

10. Cat's Claw:

Not sourced from felines, but from a woody vine, Cat's claw has a longstanding history in traditional medicine. Several studies propose its potential anticancer effects by bolstering the immune system and impeding the proliferation of cancer cells.

Quick Notes:

Consult the Pros: Before delving into herbal remedies, it's crucial to consult your healthcare team. They possess the expertise to advise you on which approaches align best with your treatment plan.

One Size Doesn't Fit All: Just because a remedy was effective for someone else doesn't guarantee the same results for you. It's essential to recognize that each person's body responds differently, so individual experiences may vary.

Not a Replacement: These herbs serve as supportive allies rather than primary protagonists. They can enhance your conventional treatments but should not be viewed as substitutes. It's important to bear this in mind.

13

The power of green tea

Let's delve into the intriguing world of green tea and its possible role as a superhero battling against cancer.

Origins of Green Tea:

Imagine this – green tea, an age-old potion originating from China. It's more than just a comforting beverage; it's enriched with compounds that researchers are investigating for their potential health benefits.

The Power of Polyphenols:

The secret lies within polyphenols, particularly catechins. These tiny defenders act as antioxidants, diligently combating free radicals that might otherwise cause cellular harm and, as you've probably guessed, increase the risk of cancer.

Anti-Cancer Potential:

This is where it gets intriguing. Research suggests that green tea could act as a gatekeeper against cancer growth. Catechins, notably EGCG, appear to possess the ability to interfere with the mechanisms that cancer cells depend on for their survival.

Guarding Against DNA Damage:

Green tea could serve as your DNA's protector. By shielding against oxidative damage, it acts as a barrier, preventing mutations that could initiate cancer development.

Slowing Tumor Growth:

Green tea extracts could potentially slow down tumor growth like a gentle reminder to the speeding train, urging it to ease off and proceed with caution.

Targeting Multiple Cancers:

Green tea appears to be versatile, playing various roles in the cancer scenario across different types such as breast, prostate, lung, colorectal, and more.

Promoting Cancer Cell Death:

Here's the fascinating aspect: green tea could be signaling to cancer cells that their time is up, acting like a switch that says, "Alright, it's time to wrap things up."

Inhibiting Angiogenesis:

Cancers rely on angiogenesis, the formation of new blood vessels, to thrive. The catechins in green tea intervene, halting the process and preventing tumors from getting the blood supply they need.

Enhancing the Immune System

Green tea goes beyond direct combat; it also energizes your immune system. According to some studies, it acts as a motivator for your immune cells, priming them to defend against cancer and other threats.

Managing Treatment Side Effects

Outside of the cancer fight itself, green tea could serve as a helpful ally during treatments, potentially providing some relief by assisting in the management of challenging side effects.

Cautions and Considerations

However, it's essential to remember that green tea isn't a cure-all solution. Individual responses can differ, and excessive consumption may not be advisable. Consistently incorporating moderate amounts into your routine may yield better results than occasional consumption. In the realm of combating cancer, green tea emerges as a promising ally, providing a blend of antioxidants and compounds that disrupt cancer's progression. Here's to embracing hope

and well-being with each sip of green tea.
Cheers!

14

Important of Raw foods

Let's delve into the remarkable nutritional benefits of embracing raw and whole foods – those genuine, unprocessed ingredients sourced directly from nature.

Pure, Unaltered Goodness:
Consider raw and whole foods as nature's unadulterated contribution to your meals. They're akin to the celebrities of nutrition, retaining all their natural goodness – brimming with vitamins, minerals, and antioxidants that your body craves.

Rich in Essential Nutrients:
Imagine a colorful array of fresh fruits, crunchy vegetables, and hearty grains. This is the cast of characters in raw and whole foods, providing the

vital nutrients necessary for everything from robust bones to a resilient immune system.

Enzymatic Magic:

One fascinating aspect of raw foods is that they contain their own enzymes. These enzymes act as digestive superheroes, aiding your body in breaking down food and enhancing the efficiency of digestion.

Antioxidant Heaven:

Raw fruits and vegetables are akin to an antioxidant celebration. They are dedicated to combating oxidative stress, a form of stress that can disrupt your cells and contribute to conditions such as cancer and premature aging.

Fiber Boost:

Raw and whole foods excel as champions of fiber. Packed with dietary fiber, they are the long-awaited ally of your digestive system. Fiber promotes regular bowel movements and maintains gut health by ensuring smooth digestion.

Micronutrient Marvels:
Every mouthful of raw and whole foods is a voyage through a realm of vitamins and minerals. Whether it's the vitamin C found in citrus fruits or the potassium abundant in bananas, these foods offer a rich array of micronutrients to enhance your nutritional intake.

Blood Sugar Balance:
Opting for whole foods, particularly those with a low glycemic index, aids in maintaining stable blood sugar levels. This approach provides a consistent energy source, steering clear of the fluctuations often associated with processed or refined foods.

Healthy Fats Source:

Nuts, seeds, and avocados play a vital role as sources of healthy fats, often overlooked. They promote heart health, aid in nutrient absorption, and contribute to overall well-being, offering your body the beneficial fats it needs.

Reduced Processing Risks:

Opting for raw and whole foods minimizes the potential hazards linked with food processing. It streamlines the journey from the farm to your table, lessening exposure to additives, preservatives, and other undesirable substances.

Satiety and Weight Management:

Have you ever experienced that feeling of fullness and satisfaction after enjoying a nourishing salad or a bowl of fresh fruit? That's the wonder of whole foods. With their high fiber content and rich nutrient profile, they support weight management by helping you feel satiated and balanced, all without any sense of deprivation.

Remember the Variety:
The key to maximizing the nutritional benefits of raw and whole foods lies in diversity. Embrace the spectrum of colors, textures, and varieties available. Whether you're savoring the crispness of vegetables, the sweetness of fruits, or the richness of avocados, each food offers its distinct array of nutrients, enriching your diet with a wide range of healthful properties.

In a landscape where convenience often steals the show, raw and whole foods stand out as the unsung champions of nutrition. They provide a direct route to well-being and energy, encouraging you to relish the wholesome bounty of nature, one delightful taste at a time. Here's to fueling your body with genuine goodness!

15

Blackened Meat or Not?

Let's simplify the link between meat and cancer without diving into complex scientific terms, focusing on what the research reveals and how it impacts our well-being.

When we talk about traditional red meats such as beef, lamb, and pork, along with processed meats like bacon and sausages, studies suggest that consuming these regularly might heighten the risk of specific cancers.

Here's where it gets intriguing: Cooking meat at high temperatures, particularly through grilling or smoking, can generate compounds known as HCAs and PAHs. These substances act as the antagonists in our meat-related narrative and could potentially contribute to the elevated cancer risk we're discussing.

Colorectal cancer takes center stage in the meat discussion. Several studies suggest that indulging in red and processed meats regularly may elevate the risk of colorectal cancer. Although the exact mechanism remains unclear, these compounds could potentially disrupt colon cell function.

However, before you bid farewell to steak forever, moderation appears to be key. Some research indicates that maintaining a balanced and moderate intake of meat, particularly lean varieties, may not pose the same risks. It's not an all-or-nothing scenario.

Meat provides essential nutrients like protein, iron, zinc, and B-vitamins. Completely eliminating it from your diet could lead to missing out on these vital nutrients. Therefore, it's essential to find a middle ground that satisfies our bodies' nutritional needs while minimizing potential risks.

The meat-cancer connection is influenced by various individual factors such as genetics, lifestyle choices, and dietary habits. What poses a risk for one person may not necessarily have the same impact on another individual, making it akin to a personalized health puzzle.

If you're feeling wary about your burger now, there's no need to panic – there are alternatives and adjustments you can make. Opting for leaner cuts of meat, incorporating plant-based protein sources, and choosing cooking methods that minimize the formation of potentially harmful compounds can all be part of a proactive approach.

Processed meats have raised concerns among major health organizations. The World Health

Organization (WHO) categorizes them as Group 1 carcinogens, indicating substantial evidence linking them to cancer. Therefore, it might be wise to reserve indulging in items like bacon for special occasions.

Remember, it's essential to consider the broader context, not just focusing on meat alone but looking at the entire spectrum of your diet. A well-balanced eating plan that includes a variety of foods like fruits, vegetables, whole grains, and lean proteins is key to maintaining overall health. It's like orchestrating a symphony of nutrients that keeps our bodies in harmony and singing a healthy tune.

The conversation around meat and its potential link to cancer is ongoing and continually evolving as new research emerges. Staying informed and consulting with healthcare professionals can provide valuable guidance as you navigate the complexities of dietary choices and their potential impact on health.

16

The Power of Spirituality

Let's delve into the profound significance of spirituality in the process of healing from cancer. It transcends mere physical treatment, offering solace to the soul and fortitude in the immaterial dimensions of existence.

Imagine spirituality as a steadfast beacon for individuals grappling with cancer. It serves as a bastion of emotional strength, a soothing force that imparts hope and connectivity beyond the confines of conventional medicine. Amidst the tempest of diagnosis and treatment, this emotional fortitude serves as a lifeline.

Have you ever experienced a profound sense of purpose that transcends the mundane routines of daily life? Spirituality imbues the healing journey with that essence. It's more than just combatting an illness; it involves grasping the intricacies of existence, illness, and one's distinct purpose. This deeper significance serves as a motivating force, propelling individuals to persevere and emerge victorious.

Spirituality isn't merely a passive observer; it actively participates in coping mechanisms. Whether through prayer, meditation, or engagement in spiritual communities, it offers a framework for navigating the tumultuous emotions that accompany a cancer diagnosis. It becomes the steadfast support during challenging times.

We're well aware that stress isn't an ally, particularly during cancer treatment. Spirituality emerges as a valuable stress-reliever. Through rituals such as prayer or meditation, it establishes a sanctuary for inner calm. It functions akin to a pause button, enabling individuals to catch their breath and discover serenity amid the turmoil.

There's a unique quality to the camaraderie found within a spiritual community. It serves as a hub of connection, empathy, and collective experiences. Whether within a religious institution or through personal spiritual beliefs, this network of support becomes an invaluable source of solace and belonging.

Confronting cancer can feel like venturing into unknown territory. Spirituality serves as a guiding compass in such moments. It empowers individuals, enabling them to actively shape their healing journey by aligning their decisions with their spiritual beliefs. It emphasizes taking an engaged stance rather than being a passive bystander.

Have you experienced the transformative influence of a positive mindset? Spirituality delves into the mind-body connection, acknowledging practices like meditation or mindfulness as more than just mental relaxation techniques. They contribute to holistic well-being, recognizing the interconnectedness of mental and physical health.

Amidst the challenges of cancer, hope emerges as a vital lifeline. Spirituality imbues a deep sense of hope and positivity, whether through belief in a higher power or a broader spiritual understanding, igniting optimism and a healing-oriented mindset even in the darkest times.

Spirituality isn't merely about enduring; it's about embracing life to the fullest extent. It's been associated with an improved quality of life for individuals grappling with cancer, extending beyond physical health to encompass emotional well-being, pain management, and the ability to find joy amidst adversity.

Consider spirituality as a foundational element within the realm of holistic healing. It resonates with the notion that true well-being entails addressing not only the physical aspects but also the spiritual and emotional dimensions. It complements the medical journey by offering a broader perspective.

Thus, in the process of recovering from cancer, spirituality emerges as an invisible guiding presence, a supportive ally in the background, providing fortitude, endurance, and a deep wellspring of optimism. It serves as a testament to the understanding that healing encompasses various interconnected elements, where the nurturing of the soul holds equal significance alongside medical interventions and therapies.

Conclusion

In In the concluding sections of "Prevent and Beat Cancer," we find ourselves at the intersection of scientific knowledge and spiritual insight, where the process of healing extends beyond the boundaries of traditional understanding. It has been a voyage through the complex interplay of mind, body, and spirit, where every element contributes to narratives of strength, optimism, and profound revelations.

A Symphony of Healing:
Picture this book as a symphony, where each chapter contributes a distinctive note to the harmony of your journey toward healing. From the clinical realms of medical interventions to the tranquil realms of spirituality, we've crafted a symphonic fusion that echoes the essence of comprehensive healing.

Dancing with Uncertainty:

In the intricate choreography of confronting cancer, uncertainty emerges as an unavoidable companion. However, equipped with the understanding that healing extends beyond medical procedures, we gracefully navigated through the uncharted territories. It's not about evading the tempest, but rather about mastering the art of dancing amidst adversity—a symbolic gesture of embracing life's trials with fortitude and resilience.

Whispers of Spirituality:

Amidst the gentle whispers of spirituality, we unearthed a reservoir of resilience that surpasses the bounds of the tangible. It emerged as a steadfast ally, an illuminating presence amidst darkness, leading us through the maze of emotions, providing comfort, and infusing a deeper sense of meaning that transcends mere medical prognosis.

Beyond Surviving, Thriving:
This voyage isn't just about enduring; it's an invitation to flourish despite challenges. Embracing the holistic perspective urges us to reimagine the essence of genuine living, discovering happiness in the simplest of joys, and cherishing life's splendor even amidst illness. It's a tribute to resilience and the indomitable human essence.

Empowerment in Choices:
As we conclude this segment, keep in mind that you wield the quill for your tale. The holistic route enables you to make decisions aligned with your convictions and principles. It's about seizing command over your narrative, embracing the role of the author in your journey to

wellness, and traversing unfamiliar territories guided by a spiritual compass.

The Unfinished Story:
Our voyage within these lines marks merely a single passage in the larger narrative of your existence. The tale remains incomplete, with unwritten pages eagerly anticipating the imprints of your encounters, victories, and instances of deep insight. It beckons you to persist in the expedition, equipped with the understanding that healing embodies a fluid, perpetual storyline.

As we conclude this guide, let the curtain descend not on a conclusion but on a fresh commencement. May the insights gleaned resonate within you, and may the wisdom gained illuminate your onward journey. As the closing chords of this symphony fade away, recall that your narrative is a work of art, showcasing the resilience of the human soul and the profound impact of holistic wellness. May your path be adorned with healing, optimism, and the steadfast conviction that life, truly, is a melody worth cherishing.

Review

Dear Reader,

I trust this message finds you in good spirits. I'm reaching out to extend my heartfelt thanks for opting to delve into this book. It's been an enriching experience, and my earnest wish is that you found the book enlightening and worthwhile.

As a writer, your input holds significant value for me. I would deeply appreciate it if you could spare a moment to provide your thoughts and reflections by leaving a review on the platform where you obtained the book.

Your review offers both invaluable insights for me and assists potential readers in discovering the book's relevance to their interests and needs. Whether you share a brief comment or a comprehensive reflection, your honest feedback is immensely valued.

Thank you once more for accompanying me on this journey. I eagerly anticipate your feedback and deeply value the time and thoughtfulness you dedicate to it.

Warm regards,

Dr Mark Rainey